COMPLETE GUIDE TO ARTHROSCOPIC SURGERY

Advanced Techniques, Minimally Invasive Procedures, Rehabilitation Protocols, And Recovery Strategies For Orthopedic Joint Conditions

DR. BRUNO HORAN

Copyright © 2023 by Dr. Bruno Horan

All rights reserved. Except for brief quotations embodied in critical reviews and certain other noncommercial uses permitted by copyright law, no part of this publication may be reproduced, distributed, or transmitted in any form or by any means, Including photocopying, recording, or other electronic or mechanical methods, without the prior written permission of the publisher.

Disclaimer:

The information provided in this book, is intended for general informational purposes only and should not be considered as professional advice.

The author has made every effort to ensure the accuracy of the information presented. However, readers are advised to consult with a qualified healthcare professional before attempting any herbal remedies or making significant changes to their wellness routine. Individual health conditions vary, and what may be suitable for one person may not be appropriate for another.

It is important to note that the author is not in any endorsement deal, partnership, or affiliation with any organization, brand, or company mentioned in this book. Any references to specific products or services are based on the author's personal experience or general knowledge and do not imply an endorsement or promotion of those products or services

Contents

CHAPTER ONE 11
  ANATOMICAL FOUNDATIONS 11
    Synopsis Of Joint Anatomy 11
    Knowing About Tendons And Ligaments 12
    Surrounding Muscles Of Joints 14
    Typical Joint Pathologies 15

CHAPTER TWO 17
  GUIDELINES FOR ARTHROSCOPY: 17
    Conditions That Arthroscopic Surgery Can Treat . 18
    Criteria For Patient Evaluation 21
    Using Imaging Methods In Arthroscopy 22
    Early Intervention's Advantages 23

CHAPTER THREE 27
  SURGICAL METHODS 27
    Instrumentation And Portals 28
    Managing Fluids During Arthroscopy 29
    Step-By-Step Operative Techniques 30

CHAPTER FOUR 33
  CARE AFTER POSTOPERATION 33

- Protocols For Recovery Rooms 33
- Techniques For Pain Management 34
- Keeping An Eye Out For Complications 36
- Going Back To Our Regular Activities 37

CHAPTER FIVE 39
COMMON PRACTICE 39
- Arthroscopy Of The Knee: ACL Reconstruction ... 39
- Repair Of The Rotator Cuff By Shoulder Arthroscopy 41
- Hip Arthroscopy: Ligament Restoration 42
- Ankle Arthroscopy: Excision Of Loose Bodies 43
- Osteochondritis Dissecans Treatment With Elbow Arthroscopy 45

CHAPTER SIX 47
ARTHROSCOPIC SURGERY ADVANCES 47
- New Developments In Arthroscopy 47
- Minimally Adverse Methods 48
- AUTOMATION IN ARTHROSCOPIC SURGERY 49
- Upcoming Developments And Trends 50

CHAPTER SEVEN 53

COMMUNICATION AND EDUCATION OF PATIENTS 53
- Taking Care Of Patient Expectations 54
- Process Of Informed Consent 55
- Giving Instructions Following Surgery 56
- Resolving Patient Issues And Inquiries 57

CHAPTER EIGHT 59
FAQS AND REGULAR QUESTIONS 59
- How Long Does It Take To Recover From Arthroscopic Surgery 59
- After Arthroscopic Surgery, Can I Drive? 60
- When Can I Start Playing Sports Or Getting Physical Again? 61
- What Possible Dangers Are Associated With Arthroscopy? 62
- After Surgery, Are There Any Dietary Restrictions? 63

CONCERNING THIS BOOK

"Arthroscopic Surgery" is a vital tool that explores the complex realm of minimally invasive joint surgery and offers a thorough manual for both experienced professionals and beginners in the field.

Its thorough examination begins with a basis in the development and history of arthroscopic procedures, shedding light on how these innovations have improved patient outcomes.

The book describes the risks and benefits of arthroscopic surgery in detail, ensuring that medical professionals are aware of the trade-off between probable consequences and benefits.

For every surgical professional, understanding the fundamentals of anatomy is essential, and this is covered in great detail throughout the book.

Joint anatomy, ligaments, tendons, cartilage, and surrounding muscles are all carefully covered, providing the comprehensive knowledge required for accurate surgical procedures. Common joint diseases are also covered in this section, which lays the groundwork for comprehending the precise reasons for arthroscopy.

A detailed analysis is conducted of the practical issues of doing arthroscopic surgery. This covers the necessary planning, such as choosing the right instruments and equipment, comprehending the standards for patient evaluation, and making efficient use of imaging methods.

The part on surgical techniques provides comprehensive instructions on how to manage fluids, position patients, choose anesthetic, and follow step-by-step protocols to guarantee positive results.

Another crucial area of attention is postoperative care, which includes thorough guidelines for managing pain, recovery room techniques, and exercise regimens. Ensuring a quick and safe recovery lowers the chance of complications and makes it easier for patients to resume their regular activities.

Particular popular procedures are also covered, offering particular insights into these often-done surgeries. These procedures include labral repair, rotator cuff repair, and ACL reconstruction.

The book offers techniques to avoid and manage problems like infection, nerve and vascular damage, and anesthesia-related adverse responses. It doesn't hold back when discussing complications and risk management.

Furthermore, it explores cutting-edge technologies, robots, minimally invasive procedures, and biological agents that are poised to transform the field of arthroscopic surgery.

To make sure that patients are informed and that their expectations are appropriately handled,

"Arthroscopic Surgery" places a strong emphasis on patient education and communication.

This covers guidelines for postoperative care, informed consent procedures, and preoperative counseling. The book is a priceless tool for improving patient care and surgical excellence because it ends with a section that answers often-asked questions and common concerns.

CHAPTER ONE

ANATOMICAL FOUNDATIONS

Synopsis Of Joint Anatomy

The places where two or more bones come together to form joints allow for movement and mechanical support. The human body is made up of various joint types that are distinguished by their structural makeup and range of motion. The most prevalent kind of joints are synovial ones, which include the hip, knee, and shoulder joints. The fluid-filled synovial cavity in these joints allows for smoother motion and less friction. Articular cartilage, a smooth, white layer that lowers friction and absorbs stress, covers the bones in synovial joints.

Fibrous joints, like the sutures in the skull, are joined by extensive connective tissue and are immobile. Cartilaginous joints, such as those that link the vertebrae in the spine, are cartilaginous structures that can move slightly. Comprehending the fundamental varieties of joints facilitates the understanding of the intricate mechanisms that enable mobility and reinforces the significance of arthroscopic surgery in the diagnosis and management of joint disorders.

Knowing About Tendons And Ligaments

Important parts of the musculoskeletal system that promote mobility and provide stability are tendons and ligaments. Ligaments, which connect bones to other bones at joints, are strong, flexible bands of connective tissue. They aid in guiding appropriate mobility and preserving joint stability. For example, the knee's anterior cruciate ligament (ACL) is crucial for maintaining joint stability when running and jumping.

Conversely, the tendon attaches muscles to bones. They allow movement by transferring the force produced by muscles to the skeleton. For example, the Achilles tendon, which connects the calf muscles to the heel bone, is essential for sprinting, jumping, and walking. Due to degenerative changes, trauma, or misuse, ligaments and tendons can sustain damage that frequently necessitates surgery to return to normal function.

Cartilage: Composition and Purpose

Cartilage is a hard and flexible connective tissue that is present in the nose, ears, joints, and rib cage, among other regions of the body. The extremities of bones in joints are covered in articular cartilage, which facilitates low-friction movement by offering a smooth, lubricated surface for articulation. In addition, it serves as a cushion, absorbing impacts from exercises like jogging and walking.

Because cartilage is avascular—that is, devoid of blood vessels—its capacity to mend injury is restricted. Damage to the cartilage can cause discomfort, edema, and decreased movement. Osteoarthritis is a common cartilage problem characterized by progressive cartilage loss that causes stiffness and pain in the joints. These issues can be resolved with arthroscopic surgery, which restores joint function by replacing or repairing damaged cartilage.

Surrounding Muscles Of Joints

Muscles are essential for the stability and movement of joints. The muscles that surround each joint contract and relax to create mobility.

For instance, the supraspinatus, infraspinatus, teres minor, and subscapularis are among the rotator cuff muscles that surround the shoulder joint. Together, these muscles support the shoulder and enable a variety of motions, including lifting and rotating the arm.

Likewise, the hamstrings and quadriceps support the knee joint. The hamstrings, which are found at the rear of the thigh, flex the knee, whereas the quadriceps, which are found at the front of the thigh, extend it. For joints to remain healthy and function properly, these muscles must remain flexible and strong. These muscles can become weak or injured, which increases the risk of injuries and causes joint instability.

Typical Joint Pathologies

Disorders or diseases that affect the joints and cause pain, swelling, or dysfunction are referred to as joint pathologies.

Osteoarthritis, a degenerative disorder where the cartilage that cushions the ends of bones breaks down over time, producing pain and stiffness, is one of the most frequent joint pathologies.

An inflammatory condition called rheumatoid arthritis results in inflammation of the joint lining, which in turn produces pain and swelling.

Additional frequent joint disorders include tendonitis, an inflammation of the tendons sometimes brought on by overuse, and ligament tears, such as ACL injuries in the knee.

Athletes frequently sustain meniscus tears, which are caused by injury to the knee's cartilage. These diseases are commonly diagnosed and treated using arthroscopic surgery, which offers a less invasive means of removing or repairing damaged tissue and restoring joint function.

CHAPTER TWO

GUIDELINES FOR ARTHROSCOPY:

Arthroscopy is recommended for both therapeutic and diagnostic uses. When non-invasive imaging tests like X-rays or MRIs are insufficient in explaining a patient's joint pain, swelling, or instability, this minimally invasive surgical approach is usually taken into consideration.

Patients who continue to experience joint pain after trying conservative measures including medication, physical therapy, and rest are good candidates for arthroscopy.

Evaluation and treatment of meniscal tears, ligament injuries, cartilage loss, and synovial problems in joints such as the knee, shoulder, elbow, ankle, and wrist are common indications.

Additionally, synovectomy, debridement of joint surfaces, and the removal of loose bodies may be indicated by arthroscopy. It's also utilized to diagnose inflammation and pain in the joints that cannot be explained when other techniques have not yielded a definitive diagnosis.

Conditions That Arthroscopic Surgery Can Treat

Because of its versatility, arthroscopic surgery can treat a variety of joint diseases. Conditions that are frequently addressed include:

Meniscal Tears: Knee meniscus tears are repaired or removed.

Ligament Injuries: Rebuilding or mending of ligaments, such as the knee's ACL.

Cartilage Damage: Restoring smooth joint surfaces requires treating osteochondral defects or cartilage lesions.

Repair of damaged shoulder tendons is known as rotator cuff tears.

Removal of bone spurs or inflammatory tissue-producing impingement is the treatment for shoulder impingement syndrome.

Cleaning of contaminated tissue and synovial fluid in cases of joint infections.

Elimination of inflammatory synovial tissue causes synovitis.

Removal of bone or cartilage pieces that are floating within the joint area is known as "loose bodies."

In addition to offering alleviation and better function, arthroscopy is useful in the treatment of bursitis, labral tears in the hip or shoulder, and ankle impingement syndromes.

Comparing Therapeutic and Diagnostic Arthroscopy

A diagnostic arthroscopy is a procedure used to look into a joint to determine what is causing symptoms like pain, edema, or instability.

It entails making tiny incisions in the joint to insert an arthroscope, a thin, flexible tube equipped with a camera.

When non-invasive techniques are unsatisfactory, this gives the surgeon real-time access to the internal structures of the joint, enabling an accurate diagnosis.

Conversely, therapeutic arthroscopy includes surgical treatment in addition to the same basic diagnostic procedures.

The surgeon can undertake treatments to repair or remove damaged tissue, reconstruct ligaments, or smooth down rough cartilage once the cause of the joint problem has been determined.

Because of these two advantages, arthroscopy is a highly successful diagnostic and therapeutic tool for joint problems.

Criteria For Patient Evaluation

Choosing the best candidates for an arthroscopy requires a careful assessment of the patient. Among the requirements are:

History and Physical Examination: A thorough medical history is obtained, and the afflicted joint is the main focus of the physical examination.

Individuals who are non-responsive to conservative treatment include those who have not responded well to drugs, injections, physical therapy, or lifestyle changes.

Continuous pain, edema, instability, or mechanical symptoms like locking or clicking in the joint are examples of persistent symptoms.

Imaging Research:

preliminary imaging tests (MRI, CT, and X-rays) that point to the possibility of an arthroscopic procedure to treat intra-articular disease.

General Health: A state of overall well-being that guarantees the patient can safely undergo anesthesia and surgery.

The patient's activity level, expectations, and capacity to engage in postoperative therapy are all taken into account during the evaluation.

Using Imaging Methods In Arthroscopy

Imaging is essential to the planning and performance of arthroscopic surgery. Techniques for preoperative imaging consist of:

X-rays: Give a general picture of bone structure, joint alignment, and the presence of fractures or arthritis.

Pre-operative planning is greatly aided by magnetic resonance imaging (MRI), which provides finely detailed images of soft tissues such as ligaments, cartilage, menisci, and synovium.

Less commonly used yet capable of producing precise images of bone and joint structures, computed tomography (CT) scans are especially helpful in cases with complicated joint anatomy or bone injuries.

Ultrasound: Occasionally used to image soft tissue structures in real-time, especially the shoulder and other joints that are easily accessible.

During arthroscopy, intraoperative imaging, such as fluoroscopy, can also be utilized to guide surgical instruments and verify the precision of procedures like joint alignment or hardware implantation.

Early Intervention's Advantages

Significant advantages can be obtained via arthroscopic surgery at an early stage, such as:

Reduced Joint Damage: Prompt intervention can stop additional joint structural degradation, maintaining function and lowering the need for later, more intrusive procedures.

Faster Recovery: Patients can resume regular activities and work sooner after arthroscopy since it is less intrusive than open surgery and usually requires less time to recover.

Pain Relief: Early surgical surgery can enhance joint function and reduce pain more quickly, which will improve the patient's quality of life.

Reduced Risk of Complications: Treating joint problems at an early stage can help lower the chance of long-term joint damage complications including arthritis and chronic pain.

superior Results: Early intervention for joint diseases or injuries frequently produces superior long-term results, including greater success and patient satisfaction rates.

Arthroscopy is a vital tool in the therapy of musculoskeletal disorders since it can simultaneously identify and cure joint abnormalities, highlighting the significance of early, proactive medical action.

CHAPTER THREE

SURGICAL METHODS

Options for Anesthesia During Arthroscopic Surgery

Selecting the right anesthetic to be used is a critical decision to make before beginning arthroscopic surgery.

General anesthesia, regional anesthesia, and local anesthesia are the main three alternatives. General anesthesia is appropriate for lengthier or more complicated surgeries since it keeps the patient unconscious throughout the process. With the help of nerve blocks, regional anesthesia numbs a particular area of the body, allowing the patient to stay awake while experiencing pain relief.

Usually used for simple procedures or in conjunction with sedation, local anesthesia entails injecting medicine to numb only the operative site.

Putting the Patient in Position

For the best possible access to the joint and to ensure the patient's safety and comfort throughout the process, proper patient placement is essential. On the operating table, the patient is often placed on their back, with the operative limb suitably exposed and reachable.

Different positions may be used, depending on the joint being operated on. To make it easier to access the joint space during a knee arthroscopy, for instance, the patient's leg may be placed in a leg holder or inside a specialized traction device. Bony prominences are carefully padded, and the patient's position is carefully monitored to ensure proper blood flow and ventilation.

Instrumentation And Portals

Small incisions around the joint are called portals, through which the arthroscope and other surgical tools are inserted. The surgeon can view and work with the joint's internal structures through these ports. The surgeon's discretion and the particular procedure being performed determine the number and location of portals. In most cases, two or four portals are employed during arthroscopy procedures. After the portals are created, specialized tools are introduced through them to carry out the required surgical procedures. These tools include the arthroscope, graspers, scissors, shavers, and probes.

Managing Fluids During Arthroscopy

A sterile saline solution is continuously pushed into the joint during arthroscopy to clear debris, provide space, and improve vision. Maintaining a clear surgical area and reducing the possibility of problems like heat injury and fluid extravasation are made possible by this fluid management system.

Throughout the process, the fluid's pressure and flow rate are closely controlled to guarantee that the joint is distended as much as possible without limiting circulation or producing excessive edema. After the procedure, the extra fluid is removed from the joint and any bleeding is stopped before the portals are closed.

Step-By-Step Operative Techniques

Regardless of the precise treatment being carried out, arthroscopic surgery usually follows a methodical set of stages.

Once the patient is in the correct posture and has received anesthesia, the surgeon starts by creating portals around the joint with tiny incisions. The internal structures of the joint are then visible on a display once the arthroscope is introduced through one of these ports.

The surgeon continuously evaluates the state and function of the joint while executing the necessary debridement or reconstruction using specialized devices inserted through the other portals.

The surgeon may move the joint during the process to assess stability, range of motion, and general function.

The instruments are taken out and the portals are sealed with adhesive strips or sutures after the surgical goals are met. Before being released from the hospital, the patient is attentively watched for any indications of difficulties and is given post-operative care instructions.

CHAPTER FOUR

CARE AFTER POSTOPERATION

Protocols For Recovery Rooms

The initial postoperative phase following arthroscopic surgery is critical to a successful recovery. Usually, patients are brought to a special recovery area where they are closely observed by healthcare providers. Vital signs including blood pressure, oxygen saturation, and heart rate are continuously watched in this regulated environment to guarantee stability.

Patients may also be given drugs to control pain and nausea as well as intravenous fluids to stay hydrated. Because anesthetic often causes patients to feel drowsy or confused just after surgery, they must get plenty of rest under close monitoring until they are completely conscious and alert.

Depending on how each person reacts to the surgery and anesthesia, the amount of time spent in the recovery room can change. The patient may be moved to a regular hospital room or released home with the necessary instructions for continued recovery if they are judged stable and their vital signs are within normal ranges.

Techniques For Pain Management

One of the most important aspects of postoperative treatment after arthroscopic surgery is effective pain management. Even though some soreness is inevitable following any surgical operation, pain management is crucial to fostering healing and facilitating recovery.

There are other ways to control pain, such as taking oral medications like NSAIDs (nonsteroidal anti-inflammatory drugs) or opioids (opioids) for more severe cases. To further relieve specific pain at the surgery site, local anesthetics may also be used.

Non-pharmacological methods including cold therapy, elevating the afflicted limb, and light massage may also assist lessen pain and swelling in addition to pharmaceutical interventions. To make necessary modifications to their pain management strategy, patients must be able to honestly discuss their pain levels with their healthcare providers.

Exercises for Rehabilitation

After arthroscopic surgery, rehabilitation activities are essential for regaining function and mobility. Physical therapists usually prescribe these exercises, which are customized to meet the demands of each patient and the particular procedure carried out.

To avoid stiffness and preserve flexibility in the injured joint, mild range-of-motion exercises might be the major focus during the early phases of healing. Exercises to enhance stability and strengthen the surrounding muscles may be added as the healing process moves forward.

Patients are advised to follow their recommended workout program exactly since consistency is essential to getting the best results. To prevent harm or setbacks in the healing process, it is imperative to proceed cautiously and refrain from exerting excessive force.

Keeping An Eye Out For Complications

Even though arthroscopic surgery is usually seen to be safe, problems can occasionally occur in the aftermath. Infection, severe bleeding, blood clots, and negative anesthetic or drug reactions are examples of common consequences.

Patients are usually told to keep an eye out for symptoms like fever, shortness of breath, chest pain, growing pain, redness, swelling, or discharge at the surgery site to monitor for these potential consequences. Any worrisome symptoms should be brought to the attention of a healthcare professional right once for additional assessment and treatment.

Healthcare professionals will have routine follow-up appointments in addition to self-monitoring to evaluate the patient's progress, keep an eye out for any indications of difficulties, and modify the treatment plan as needed.

Going Back To Our Regular Activities

After arthroscopic surgery, a crucial part of postoperative care is gradually returning to regular activities. Although it's understandable to want things to get back to normal, you should take caution and adhere to any instructions given by the medical staff.

Patients may need to limit activities that put too much stress on the surgical site or interfere with healing during the early phases of recovery. These limitations could apply to lifting large things, playing sports or other high-impact activities, or standing or walking for extended periods.

Patients can progressively increase their degree of exercise and return to their regular daily routines as their recovery advances and healing milestones are met. But, it's crucial to pay attention to your body and refrain from exerting too much pressure on oneself too soon, as this may impede healing or raise the possibility of problems.

In general, the process of getting back to your regular activities should be gradual and steady, guided by your healthcare provider's suggestions. You can increase your chances of a speedy recovery and a return to an active, healthy lifestyle by adhering to these recommendations and practicing patience with yourself.

CHAPTER FIVE
COMMON PRACTICE

Arthroscopy Of The Knee: ACL Reconstruction

A minimally invasive surgical technique called knee arthroscopy is used to identify and address a range of knee issues.

Anterior cruciate ligament (ACL) reconstruction is a frequently performed knee arthroscopic operation. One important stabilizing ligament in the knee, the ACL, can be ripped or injured while playing sports or engaging in other physical activity.

An arthroscope, a tiny camera, is inserted by the surgeon through tiny incisions made around the knee during an ACL reconstruction. This spares them from making a huge incision and allows them to see inside the knee joint.

The injured ACL is then removed by the surgeon using tiny surgical instruments, and it is replaced with a graft created from the patient's tissue or tissue from a donor.

After being fixed in position with screws or other fixation tools, the graft will eventually blend in with the surrounding tissue to stabilize the knee joint.

The majority of ACL reconstruction procedures are done as outpatient procedures, thus patients can usually return home the same day of the procedure.

Physical therapy is typically used to strengthen the knee muscles and increase the range of motion after an ACL repair.

The recuperation process typically includes a period of rest. After surgery, the majority of patients can resume their regular activities six to nine months later; however, athletes may need more time to resume full-time sports participation.

Repair Of The Rotator Cuff By Shoulder Arthroscopy

A minimally invasive surgical technique called shoulder arthroscopy is used to identify and address a range of shoulder issues. A typical arthroscopy operation for the shoulder involves rotator cuff repair. A collection of tendons and muscles that surround the shoulder joint and aid in shoulder mobility and stability is known as the rotator cuff.

An arthroscope, a tiny camera, is inserted by the surgeon through tiny incisions made all around the shoulder during rotator cuff repair. This saves them from needing to create a huge incision to examine inside the shoulder joint. Next, the surgeon repairs any rotator cuff tears or damage with tiny surgical devices.

This could entail repairing any damaged tissue or sewing the torn tendon back together. To reduce discomfort and enhance function, the surgeon can occasionally additionally need to remove bone spurs or other material from the shoulder joint.

Patients usually need to wear a sling for a while after rotator cuff repair to protect the shoulder while it heals. To help increase shoulder strength and range of motion, physical therapy is also frequently advised. After surgery, the majority of patients can anticipate going back to their regular activities in three to six months.

Hip Arthroscopy: Ligament Restoration

A minimally invasive surgical technique called hip arthroscopy is used to identify and address a range of hip issues. Labral repair is one typical hip arthroscopy technique. A ring of cartilage called the labrum encircles the hip socket and aids in joint stability.

A tiny camera known as an arthroscope is inserted by the surgeon through tiny incisions made around the hip during labral surgery. As a result, they can view within the hip joint without making a significant cut. The labrum is then repaired by the surgeon using tiny surgical instruments if there are any tears or damage.

This can include repairing any damaged tissue or piecing the ripped labrum back together. To reduce discomfort and enhance function, the surgeon can occasionally additionally need to remove bone spurs or other abnormalities from the hip joint.

Patients usually require crutches for a while following labral surgery to remove weight from the hip as it recovers. It is also typically advised to undergo physical therapy to assist increase the hip range of motion and strength. After surgery, the majority of patients can anticipate going back to their regular activities in three to six months.

Ankle Arthroscopy: Excision Of Loose Bodies

A minimally invasive surgical technique called an ankle arthroscopy is used to identify and address a range of ankle issues. Removing loose bodies from the ankle joint is one frequent use for ankle arthroscopy. Fragments of bone or cartilage known as loose bodies can get lodged in a joint, causing discomfort and inflammation.

A tiny camera known as an arthroscope is inserted by the surgeon through tiny incisions made around the ankle during loose body removal. This spares them from making a huge incision and allows them to examine inside the ankle joint. Subsequently, the surgeon employs tiny surgical tools to extract any remaining tissues from the joint.

Patients usually require crutches for a while after loose body removal to remove weight from the injured ankle while it recovers. To enhance ankle strength and range of motion, physical treatment is also frequently advised. After surgery, the majority of patients can anticipate going back to their regular activities in two to four weeks.

Osteochondritis Dissecans Treatment With Elbow Arthroscopy

A minimally invasive surgical technique called elbow arthroscopy is used to identify and address a range of elbow issues. Osteochondritis dissecans therapy is one typical use for elbow arthroscopy. A portion of bone and cartilage in the elbow joint that has osteochondritis dissecans loses blood supply and starts to decompose.

An arthroscope, a tiny camera, is inserted by the surgeon through tiny incisions made around the elbow as part of the treatment for osteochondritis dissecans. This saves them from needing to create a huge incision to examine the elbow joint. Subsequently, the surgeon employs tiny surgical tools to eliminate the degenerated bone and cartilage and promote the formation of robust tissue.

In certain situations, the surgeon might also need to carry out other treatments, including bone grafting or microfracture, to encourage the elbow joint's recovery and stability. Patients with osteochondritis dissecans usually require a brace or splint to preserve the elbow throughout the healing process after therapy. To help increase elbow strength and range of motion, physical treatment is typically advised. After surgery, the majority of patients can anticipate going back to their regular activities in three to six months.

CHAPTER SIX

ARTHROSCOPIC SURGERY ADVANCES

Over the years, arthroscopic surgery has made great strides, completely changing the way that joint diseases and injuries are identified and handled. The development of arthroscopic techniques, which enable less intrusive operations with improved precision and efficacy, is one of the most noteworthy innovations. Orthopedic surgery has changed dramatically as a result of these developments, which now provide patients with shorter recovery times, lower risk of complications, and better results.

New Developments In Arthroscopy

The use of modern technology has proven to be highly beneficial for arthroscopy in recent times. Surgeons can make more precise diagnoses and treatment plans because of high-definition cameras, which provide them with crisp, detailed views of the inside of the joint.

Furthermore, sophisticated imaging modalities like CT and MRI scans support arthroscopic operations by offering preoperative joint assessments, helping surgeons diagnose pathology, and helping them design surgical strategies.

Minimally Adverse Methods

The less invasive aspect of arthroscopic surgery is its cornerstone. With arthroscopy, as opposed to open surgery, tiny incisions are made via which specialized tools and a camera are placed into the joint.

With the least amount of disruption to neighboring structures, these tools let surgeons see and treat problems inside the joint, such as ripped ligaments, damaged cartilage, or inflamed tissues.

Minimally invasive methods encourage quicker healing and rehabilitation in addition to lessening pain and scarring after surgery.

AUTOMATION IN ARTHROSCOPIC SURGERY

In arthroscopic surgery, robotics has changed the game by providing surgeons with unmatched precision and dexterity. With robotic-assisted arthroscopy, a surgeon's skill set is combined with robotic system capabilities to enable more control and extremely accurate motions during intricate procedures. Surgeons may accomplish more consistent results and carry out difficult procedures with greater ease by combining human talents with robotic technology. This ultimately benefits patients by improving surgical accuracy and lowering the risk of complications.

Biological Agents in Complementary Repair

Novel approaches to joint regeneration and repair have been made possible by developments in biological agents. Utilizing the body's inherent healing abilities, procedures like stem cell injections and platelet-rich plasma (PRP) therapy encourage tissue regeneration and repair. When used with arthroscopic treatments, these biologic medicines can help to improve joint function overall, decrease inflammation, and speed up the healing process. Through the utilization of biologic agents' regenerative capacity, surgeons can enhance surgical results and furnish patients with enduring alleviation from joint pain and dysfunction.

Upcoming Developments And Trends

Prospects for arthroscopic surgery appear bright, with room for more innovation and progress. Surgical efficiency and precision will be increased through ongoing improvement of current technology, such as better imaging systems and instrument design.

Furthermore, developments in virtual and augmented reality could completely transform surgical training and simulation by enabling surgeons to rehearse intricate procedures in a safe virtual setting. Furthermore, new options for joint repair may become available to patients in place of more invasive surgical procedures as a result of current research into tissue engineering and regenerative medicine. Future arthroscopic surgery is expected to provide even more advantages to patients as technology develops, reaffirming its place as the mainstay of contemporary orthopedic care.

CHAPTER SEVEN

COMMUNICATION AND EDUCATION OF PATIENTS

Communication and patient education are essential parts of the arthroscopic surgery procedure. Higher satisfaction levels and better results might result from making sure patients are aware of their procedure and actively involved in their care. The following are some efficient ways that medical practitioners can instruct and interact with patients during arthroscopic surgery:

Before Surgery

PTs should receive thorough preoperative counseling before arthroscopic surgery. This includes talking about the procedure's nature, advantages, possible drawbacks, and available treatment alternatives. In addition to answering any queries or worries the patient may have, medical professionals should take the time to thoroughly describe the surgical procedure in basic, intelligible terms. Diagrams and movies are examples of visual aids that might help improve comprehension.

Healthcare providers ought to evaluate the patient's surgical preparedness during preoperative counseling. This could entail assessing their general well-being, medication use, and any underlying medical issues that might have an impact on the result of the surgery. Patients should also be made aware of any preoperative instructions, including those regarding medication modifications and fasting needs.

Taking Care Of Patient Expectations

Controlling patient expectations is crucial to guaranteeing a satisfying surgical procedure. Realistic expectations about the results of arthroscopic surgery, including possible drawbacks and the recuperation period, should be communicated by healthcare professionals. Patients should be aware that although arthroscopic surgery is less invasive, recovery still takes time, and symptoms might not go away right away.

The secret to successfully managing expectations is open and honest communication. Patients should feel free to discuss their surgical concerns and objectives, and medical professionals should be honest in their evaluations based on their training and experience. Building confidence between the patient and the medical staff and avoiding disappointments are two benefits of setting reasonable expectations.

Process Of Informed Consent

One of the most important steps in the arthroscopic surgery procedure is getting informed consent. Before granting consent, healthcare providers must make sure that patients are fully informed about the procedure's risks, benefits, and alternatives. This entails giving thorough information about the particular dangers connected to arthroscopic surgery, like bleeding, infection, and nerve injury.

It is important to complete the informed consent procedure in a leisurely and comfortable way, giving patients enough time to raise questions and get clarifications. It is necessary to give written consent forms that summarize the main topics covered during the consent procedure. Before the procedure starts, patients should also be made aware of their ability to revoke their agreement at any moment.

Giving Instructions Following Surgery

Patients will need certain postoperative instructions following arthroscopic surgery to facilitate their recovery and reduce problems. Clear and succinct instructions on wound care, activity limitations, pain treatment, and follow-up appointments should be given by healthcare professionals. It is important to encourage patients to ask questions and get help if they need it when they are recovering.

It's critical to customize postoperative advice to each patient's unique requirements and situation. The length of time needed to recuperate and the degree of fitness required can be influenced by factors including age and the extent of the surgical treatment. Healthcare professionals can reduce the risk of problems and assist patients navigate the postoperative period with confidence by offering individualized guidance.

Resolving Patient Issues And Inquiries

Before or after arthroscopic surgery, patients may have questions or concerns that need to be addressed. Healthcare providers must establish a transparent and encouraging atmosphere that encourages patients to express their worries and ask questions. Answering questions from patients in a timely and compassionate manner helps reduce anxiety and improve the patient experience in general.

Patients should have easy access to healthcare providers before and after surgery, via phone calls, online consultations, or in-person consultations.

Quick answers to patient questions show a dedication to patient-centered care and can improve the rapport between the patient and the practitioner. Healthcare professionals can foster trust, contentment, and effective surgery outcomes by proactively addressing the questions and concerns of their patients.

CHAPTER EIGHT

FAQS AND REGULAR QUESTIONS

How Long Does It Take To Recover From Arthroscopic Surgery?

The length of recovery following arthroscopic surgery varies based on the particular joint being operated on, the degree of injury, and the general health of the patient. Patients can typically anticipate a few weeks to many months of recuperation time. In a matter of weeks, patients may resume their regular activities following modest treatments like a straightforward meniscal repair of the knee. Rehab for more intricate procedures, such as ligament restoration, may be necessary for several months.

Patients frequently have swelling and discomfort just after surgery, which can be controlled with ice packs and painkillers. To aid in the restoration of strength and range of motion, physical therapy typically starts shortly after surgery. Following a physical therapy program is essential to a full recovery. To track improvement, it's critical to pay close attention to the surgeon's instructions and show up for all follow-up appointments.

After Arthroscopic Surgery, Can I Drive?

Following arthroscopic surgery, driving may be affected by several variables, such as the type of surgery, the affected joint, and whether the patient is taking any painkillers that could make it unsafe for them to drive. Generally speaking, patients are recommended not to drive for at least 24 to 48 hours following surgery, particularly if they were sedated or were on narcotic painkillers.

Following lower extremity surgeries, such as those on the knee or ankle, driving may be prohibited for an extended amount of time. Patients need to make sure they can use the pedals in a comfortable, safe manner and stop in an emergency without experiencing any discomfort or hesitancy. It's a good idea to wait to drive until you can do so without experiencing any severe discomfort or mobility restrictions. It's crucial to discuss when it's safe to drive with your surgeon.

When Can I Start Playing Sports Or Getting Physical Again?

Following arthroscopic surgery, returning to sports or physical activity is very unique and contingent upon the particular treatment and the patient's level of rehabilitation. Patients may be able to resume modest activities in a few weeks following minor treatments, but hard lifting or high-impact sports may need a longer recovery period.

To guarantee a safe return to sports, it's imperative to adhere to an organized rehabilitation program, frequently overseen by a physical therapist. Usually, the program goes from mild range-of-motion exercises to strengthening exercises and eventually to drills tailored to a particular sport. Physicians frequently advise against participating in competitive sports until you have fully recovered your joint's strength, flexibility, and confidence. Depending on the surgery and the sport, this could take anywhere from three to six months or longer.

What Possible Dangers Are Associated With Arthroscopy?

As with any surgical technique, arthroscopy includes potential risks even though it is thought to be minimally intrusive and typically safe. Bleeding, clotting, and infection are common dangers. Damage to nearby tissues, such as blood vessels or nerves, is possible but uncommon. Additionally, some patients may have edema or stiffness in the operated joint.

The formation of a blood clot in the lung (pulmonary embolism) or leg (deep vein thrombosis) is an uncommon but serious risk. It's crucial to be aware of symptoms like shortness of breath or chest pain, as well as extreme pain, swelling, redness, or warmth in the leg, and to get medical help right away if they appear.

After Surgery, Are There Any Dietary Restrictions?

There are typically no special dietary requirements following surgery, but healing can be greatly aided by sticking to a nutritious, well-balanced diet. An adequate diet aids in the healing process and reduces inflammation. Make sure to consume an abundance of fruits, veggies, whole grains, and lean meats. It is also advised to drink a lot of water because hydration is quite important.

Patients may occasionally feel queasy and averse to food right after surgery if general anesthesia is used. Generally speaking, it's best to begin with light, easily-digested foods and work your way back to a regular diet. Include items that are easy on the stomach, like rice, toast, bananas, and applesauce, if taking painkillers causes an unsettled stomach.

Always abide by the exact dietary instructions provided by your surgeon, particularly if there are any worries about potential conflicts between certain foods and any medications you may be taking. See a doctor or nutritionist if you have any special dietary demands or restrictions so they can create a post-surgery food plan that suits your needs.

www.ingramcontent.com/pod-product-compliance
Lightning Source LLC
Chambersburg PA
CBHW071843210526
45479CB00001B/267